A GUIDE TO HEALING BACK PAIN

Strategies for Preventing, Managing, and Overcoming Chronic Back Pain

Shelby A. Nicholson, MD

Disclaimer

The information provided in this guide is for educational purposes only and should not replace professional medical advice. Always consult your healthcare provider for personalized guidance and recommendations related to your specific circumstances.

Copyright © 2023, Shelby A. Nicholson, MD.

Table of Contents

A GUIDE TO HEALING BACK PAIN

Shelby A. Nicholson, MD   5

Introduction

For millions of individuals throughout the globe, back discomfort is a common problem. It may cripple, obstruct everyday tasks, and lower one's quality of life. Finding efficient methods to treat back pain is essential for regaining comfort and functioning, whether it is brought on by bad posture, muscular strain, injury, or underlying medical disorders.

This in-depth book and guide attempt to provide you with helpful tips, doable solutions, and methodical methods to alleviate and cure your back pain. You may start along the path of pain relief, mobility restoration, and general well-being by putting the techniques covered here into practice.

Let's look at the case of John, a middle-aged guy with long-term back discomfort, to demonstrate the possibilities of these techniques. John's illness had a significant influence on his life. Simple activities like lifting shopping bags or stooping to tie his laces were excruciatingly difficult. He tried a variety of drugs, went through several procedures, and saw many physicians, but the agony continued.

After becoming desperate and frustrated, John decided to educate himself about back pain and look for alternate remedies. He came upon this thorough manual that was packed with useful tips and in-depth knowledge about treating back pain. He vowed to put the ideas presented in these pages into practice as he painstakingly digested the information with newfound optimism.

John started by talking about the aspects of his lifestyle that are causing his back discomfort. He discovered the value of keeping a good posture, working out often, and including stretches in his daily regimen. He employed stress reduction methods, made dietary adjustments, and even modified the ergonomics of his desk to improve general health.

John also looked into non-surgical procedures like physical therapy and rehabilitation and learned about the advantages of acupuncture and massage therapy. He realized the effectiveness of heat and cold treatment in easing his muscles' aches and pains and lowering inflammation. John discovered a mix of therapies that were effective for him via meticulous trial and error, offering him great relief from his ongoing back discomfort.

John's commitment and persistence paid off because he was equipped with a variety of practical tactics, acquired knowledge, and both. He was able to restore his mobility, take part in the things he formerly liked, and live life with fresh enthusiasm as his discomfort subsided over time.

John's experience is proof that back discomfort can be cured. Even though every person's experience is unique, this manual will provide you with the information and resources you need to start your own unique back pain relief journey. You too can revive and heal your back pain and reclaim a life free from the restrictions of discomfort and limits by comprehending the underlying reasons, putting preventative tactics into practice, researching different treatment alternatives, and adopting a holistic approach.

So, equipped with the information and will to beat this widespread illness and bring energy back to our lives, let's plunge into the depths of back pain treatment. Together, we will find the right way to a pain-free life, reviving our bodies and regaining our mobility.

A GUIDE TO HEALING BACK PAIN

Chapter One

Overview

People of all ages and socioeconomic levels have widespread back discomfort. It is a frequent complaint that may vary from minor aches and pains to severe, ongoing pain, often interfering with everyday activities and degrading the quality of life in general. To properly manage and get the right therapy for this illness, one must have a thorough understanding of the origins, kinds, and symptoms of back pain.

10 Importance of Addressing Back Pain

For several reasons, treating back pain is of the highest significance. You may enjoy major advantages and raise your level of well-being by putting your back's health first and taking measures to treat and prevent back discomfort. The following are some major benefits of addressing back pain:

Relieve

Finding relief from the agony and suffering brought on by the disease is one of the main reasons to treat back pain. You may reduce discomfort and improve your everyday functioning by putting the right treatment plans and lifestyle changes into place.

Increased Mobility

Back discomfort may restrict your range of motion and make it difficult for you to carry out daily tasks. By treating your back pain, you may recover mobility and go back to doing things like bending, lifting, and walking without pain or restrictions.

Enhanced Quality of Life

Back chronic pain may have a major influence on your general quality of life. Your capacity to work, engage in leisure pursuits, and take pleasure in time spent with family and friends may all be impacted. You may regain a feeling of normality and improve the quality of your life by taking care of your back and properly managing pain.

Prevention of Additional Consequences

Ignoring back discomfort or neglecting to appropriately handle it might eventually result in the emergence of more serious consequences. You may reduce the possibility of further harm or problems, such as nerve impingement or structural abnormalities, by proactively managing and treating back pain.

Increased Productivity

Both at work and at home, back discomfort may make it difficult for you to focus, concentrate, and complete activities effectively. You may increase your productivity and effectiveness in a variety of areas of your life by efficiently treating back pain.

Mental and Emotional Health

Mental and emotional health may suffer from chronic back pain, which can result in irritation, tension, worry, and even melancholy. Your mental health, stress levels, and attitude on life may all be improved by taking care of your back and finding reliable pain treatment.

Reduced Healthcare Costs

By treating back pain promptly and efficiently, you may be able to avoid the need for expensive surgical treatments or significant medical interventions. In the long term, taking preventative steps to care for your back may result in considerable financial savings.

Improved Posture and Spinal Health

Poor posture and spinal strain are frequent causes of back pain. By concentrating on taking care of your back, you may improve your posture, strengthen your supporting muscles, and support the best possible spinal health.

Recurrence Prevention

You may lessen your risk of experiencing back pain again by taking the right care of yourself and managing it properly. You may lower your chance of experiencing back pain in the future by putting preventative measures into practice, such as routine exercise, keeping a healthy weight, and using excellent ergonomics.

Overall Health

Looking after your overall health goes hand in hand with looking after your back. By putting your back health first, you may increase your physical fitness, lower your chance of developing other musculoskeletal conditions, and improve your quality of life in general.

In light of the many advantages it provides, treating back pain is essential. Living a healthy and meaningful life requires taking action to manage and avoid back pain, which has a variety of benefits ranging from pain relief and increased mobility to better quality of life and general well-being.

Chapter Two

Understanding Back Pain

Back pain is a common problem that affects many people at some time in their life. The good news is that it often doesn't result in a significant issue and could just be brought on by a little muscle or ligament strain.

As soon as you are able, it is best to remain moving and go on with your normal activities. Even if you first experience some pain and discomfort, moving around and working out won't make your back pain worse. Exercise will assist in your recovery.

The spine is one of the strongest parts of one's body, it can be referred to as the backbone or spinal column and serves as the source of the majority of our strength and flexibility.

It is made up of 24 bones, or vertebrae, placed one on top of the other. These bones are separated by discs, and the muscles and ligaments surrounding them are quite powerful. At the base of the back, the bones that make up the tailbone are also cemented together and free of discs.

On each side of the spine's spine, there are several little joints called facet joints that run from top to bottom. The spinal cord is protected by the vertebrae that it passes through.

The spinal cord connects to the brain at the base of the skull, and to the rest of the body through spaces between the vertebrae in the spine.

Ligaments, discs, joints, and other structural elements of your spine deteriorate with time. Even while the buildings are still robust, as you age, your back tends to become more rigid.

Causes of Back Pain

One or more of the following may be the cause of your back discomfort in addition to other potential causes. The spine becomes rigid from poor posture and inactivity, and muscles may become strained or injured. In addition to the conditions mentioned above, back pain has been linked to several other medical conditions. Some are listed below:

Spondylosis

As we age, the bones, discs, and ligaments of the spine may naturally deteriorate. We all go through this as we age, but it doesn't have to be a problem, and not everyone will feel uncomfortable as a consequence.

As we become older, the discs in our spines get thinner and the spaces between the vertebrae increase narrower. Little pieces of bone called osteophytes may form at the facet joints and vertebral borders. This disorder, known medically as spondylosis, is quite similar to the alterations osteoarthritis causes in other joints.

If the muscles around the spine and pelvis are strong and maintained flexible, spondylosis may not be as severe.

Sciatica

Numbness or tingling may sometimes be present, and leg discomfort may occasionally be associated with back pain. It is known as sciatica.

This results from compression or pressure on a spinal nerve. Leg pain may be the most difficult element of sciatica for most patients, and there may sometimes be no or very little back pain.

Sciatica is most often brought on by a bulging disc pressing on the nerve. Even though disc bulges are meant to facilitate simple spinal mobility, they sometimes 'catch' a nerve root and cause pain that travels down the leg and foot.

Recovery usually occurs rather quickly, although in exceptional cases it could take many months. Starting slowly with exercise will be very helpful for curing sciatica. Another smart move is to see a physiotherapist.

Spinal Stenosis

Back pain is sometimes linked to leg soreness that starts after a few minutes of walking and usually goes away quickly when you sit down. This is known as spinal stenosis. This is a potential outcome, either at birth or as people age.

Problems arise when something squeezes the nerves, which are situated in a little area in the core of the spine. Bone or ligament may compress the spinal canal, commonly known as the nerve root canal.

Although one leg may sometimes be worse than the other, both legs may exhibit symptoms. Most people find that resting and sitting down reduces their pain, but some people also get relief from their discomfort by walking a little slumped over. Similar to sciatica, the main complaint is often more leg pain than back pain.

Spinal stenosis and sciatica are often not serious conditions. However, if the symptoms drastically reduce your quality of life and cause you a lot of difficulties, you should speak with your doctor for more advice and to investigate what else could be done.

Other Elements

Other, less typical causes of back pain include:

Bone problems include infections and tumor inflammation, such that seen in ankylosing spondylitis, as well as osteoporosis, which is marked by bone loss and often accompanied by fractures.

A GUIDE TO HEALING BACK PAIN

Shelby A. Nicholson, MD   25

Chapter Three

Types of Back Pain

Depending on where it occurs, how long it lasts, and the underlying reasons, there are different forms of back pain. Here are a few prevalent forms of back pain:

Acute Back Pain

Back acute pain generally develops suddenly and lasts for a brief period, usually less than six weeks. Muscle strain, ligament sprain, or minor traumas are often the culprits. With rest, self-care techniques, and conservative treatments like painkillers, heat or cold therapy, and light exercises, acute back pain often goes away.

Chronic Back Pain

Back discomfort that persists for more than three months is referred to as chronic back pain. Even if the underlying injury or disease that caused it may have healed, the pain may have started as a result. Numerous conditions, including herniated discs, spinal stenosis, arthritis, and degenerative disc degeneration, may result in chronic back discomfort. A mix of medicine, physical therapy, exercise, and sometimes surgery is used to treat persistent back pain.

Radicular Back Pain

Sciatica is another name for radicular pain, which develops when a spinal nerve root is pinched or inflamed. The damaged nerve's route is followed by the pain as it radiates, often from the lower back down the buttock and into the leg. This kind of pain often coexists with other symptoms including numbness, tingling, or weakening of the muscles. Herniated discs, spinal stenosis, and nerve root impingement are typical causes of radicular discomfort. Painkillers, physical therapy, epidural steroid injections, and in extreme circumstances, surgery are all available as treatments.

Mechanical Back Pain

The most typical form of back pain, mechanical back pain, is caused by the muscles, ligaments, discs, and joints that make up the spine. It could be brought on by bad posture, muscular imbalances, overuse, or repeated actions. Mechanical back pain often gets better with rest and becomes worse with certain motions or activities. Physical therapy, posture correction, pain management methods, and exercises to strengthen the back and core muscles are often included in treatment plans.

Myofascial Pain Syndrome

Trigger points, which are hypersensitive knots or bands of muscle fibers, are a symptom of myofascial pain syndrome. These trigger points may convey pain to other parts of the body in addition to causing localized discomfort in the afflicted muscle. Muscle strain, injury, or overuse are all potential causes of myofascial pain syndrome. Physical therapy, stretching exercises, and relaxation methods are all possible forms of treatment.

Spinal Osteoarthritis

Degeneration of the cartilage that cushions the spine's joints causes spinal osteoarthritis, also known as degenerative joint disease or spondylosis. It often causes pain, stiffness, and joint inflammation. The problem can arise from old age, normal wear, and tear, or past accidents. Through medication, physical therapy, low-impact exercises, and lifestyle changes, treatment tries to control pain and enhance function.

It's crucial to remember that these are only basic classifications and that each person's back pain will be different in terms of severity, location, and associated symptoms. To identify the precise kind of back pain and create an effective treatment strategy, a correct diagnosis by a healthcare expert is essential.

Signs and Symptoms of Back Pain

People of all ages are susceptible to back discomfort, which may significantly influence everyday living. It may be a mild, lingering aching or a severe, incapacitating agony. Individuals may detect the issue and seek appropriate therapy by being aware of the back pain symptoms and indicators. We'll look at the many symptoms accompanying the different forms of back pain.

Dull, Aching feeling

A dull, aching feeling in the afflicted region is one of the most typical signs of back pain. This kind of discomfort is often persistent and may fluctuate over time. It is often characterized as a persistent pain that may occur both during rest and during physical exertion.

Back pain might sometimes present as a sharp, shooting ache. Commonly referred to as sciatica, this form of pain is frequently more severe and may radiate down the legs. Certain postures or motions, such as bending, lifting, or twisting, may set it off. The sciatic nerve, which passes from the lower back down to the legs, is often compressed or irritated, which results in sciatica.

Back discomfort may cause muscular tension and stiffness in the region that is being impacted. Because of this, it could be difficult to move about or carry out daily tasks. It's possible for the muscles to feel tight and to spasm, adding to the discomfort and suffering.

Limited Range of Motion

People who have back discomfort may find that their spine has a limited range of motion. Due to this, it may be difficult to bend, twist, or carry out certain motions without experiencing discomfort. Back pain often has indications of decreased flexibility and mobility.

Back discomfort may, in certain circumstances, spread to other parts of the body. For instance, lower back discomfort might radiate to the thighs, buttocks, and hips. This radiating pain may be a symptom of underlying diseases such as spinal stenosis or ruptured discs.

Back discomfort may result in numbness or tingling feelings in the afflicted region as well as down the legs. This often happens when the nerves in the spine are inflamed or squeezed, which causes radiculopathy. Weakness in the impacted regions may go along with these symptoms.

Weakness in Muscles

Long-term back pain may cause the muscles around the afflicted region to become weak. This may lead to a loss of muscular stability and strength, which may make it difficult to balance and coordinate oneself.

Postural Changes

People suffering from back pain may adopt strange postures to feel better. This might put additional stress on the spine and musculature, making the discomfort worse. Postural alterations that are frequent include hunching forward or leaning to one side.

Back Pain might Be Made Worse by Certain Activities

Some several motions or activities might make back pain worse. Lifting heavy things, spending a lot of time sitting or standing up, or participating in high-impact sports like sprinting or leaping are a few examples. Back discomfort that is brought on by certain behaviors might provide information about its underlying etiology.

Psychological Repercussions

People who have back pain may also experience psychological repercussions. The ongoing discomfort and agony might cause anger, anxiety, despair, and other negative emotions. It may impact appetite, disrupt sleep habits, and lower overall quality of life.

It's important to remember that depending on the underlying reason, the symptoms and indicators of back pain might change. Muscle strains, ligament sprains, ruptured discs, spinal stenosis, osteoarthritis, and skeletal abnormalities like scoliosis are among the common causes of back discomfort. It is best to speak with a medical expert for a precise diagnosis and a treatment strategy customized to the unique symptoms and underlying cause of the back pain.

Diagnostic Methods for Back Pain

To assess the potential cause of your back pain and develop the most effective treatment strategy, doctors employ a variety of instruments.

Health and Family Background

To ascertain if a back injury or underlying medical problem is the cause of the pain, your doctor will inquire about your medical history as well as your family's history. Among the inquiries, your doctor could ask:

What does your pain feel like? (such as acute, aching, or burning)

What part of your back is hurting the most specifically?

How long have you had the ache, and when did it start?

What were you doing when the discomfort first became apparent?

How bad or how severe is the pain?

What causes the pain to improve or worsen?

Do conditions like back pain or arthritis that cause chronic pain run in your family?

To determine the level of pain and to discuss your capacity to carry out everyday activities, your doctor may ask you to score your pain on a scale of 1 to 10.

Physique Checkup

Your doctor will probably do a physical examination, which could involve:

- Checking your posture and spine for any changes in the skeletal structure.

- Requesting that you raise or bend your legs to assess how movement impacts your discomfort.

- Testing the quickness, power, and sensitivity of your muscles.

Blood and Imaging Tests

The majority of patients do not need extra testing, however, sometimes physicians prescribe tests to either confirm or exclude a reason for your back discomfort. Your doctor could prescribe the items below.

- X-rays only display the bones and may be used to identify broken or fractured bones.

- The effects of aging.

- Changes in the alignment of the spine.

MRI (magnetic resonance imaging) utilizes energy from a strong magnet to generate signals that build a sequence of cross-sectional pictures. These photos or "slices" are evaluated by a computer to generate an image of the back. MRI may help identify injury or illness of the soft tissues, such as the discs, ligaments, and nerve roots in and around the spine.

A scanner is used in computerized axial tomography (CAT) to capture pictures of the back from various perspectives. Computer analysis of the photos yields three-dimensional views of the back. CAT scans, like MRI, aid in the diagnosis of disorders in the spinal canal and its surrounding tissues.
electrophysiological tests that assist assess the electrical activity in muscles, including electromyography or EMG. This scanning

examination helps medical professionals to know if there are any muscle and nerve issues.

Small quantities of radioactive material are used in bone scans to assist medical professionals view more details in the spine, such as fractures and infections. A probable reason for the back discomfort, such as an inflammatory or medical condition, might be found via blood testing.

Chapter Four

Prevention and Lifestyle Modifications

Back discomfort is something that we have all encountered at some point in our lives. The good news is that the pain typically subsides with a little bit of rest. You should not, however, ignore the discomfort or try to prevent it from happening again.

Back pain is a symptom, not a disease. This is your body's way of alerting you that you need to make some ergonomic changes because your posture is incorrect. Regarding your personal space, it indicates that you make some positive lifestyle changes and manage that niggling pain.

Maintaining Proper Posture

It takes more than just standing up straight to have an excellent posture. For your long-term well-being, it is essential. Regardless of whether you are moving or at rest, maintaining appropriate body alignment is essential to avoiding pain, injuries, and other health issues.

What steps should you then take?

Your body's alignment, which may be characterized as follows, determines your posture:

Your posture changes while you do activities like running, strolling, or leaning over to pick up something.

On the other hand, your posture doesn't change while you're immobile, as when you're sitting, standing, or sleeping.

It is crucial to have a straight spine in both dynamic and static settings.

The position of your spine is essential for having good posture. Your spine has three unique curves that are present naturally in the neck, mid-back, and low-back areas. Through good posture, these curves should be maintained rather than highlighted. Your head should be squarely above your shoulders, and the tops of your shoulders should be in line with your hips.

How can I stand more upright in general?

- Pay attention to your posture while doing everyday tasks like watching television, cleaning the dishes, or walking.
- Keep moving: While specific exercises may be especially helpful, any activity may help you improve your posture. They include yoga, tai chi, and other

body-awareness-focused classes. Exercises that build up the muscles in your back, stomach, and pelvis are another wise choice.

- Considering a healthy weight Weight increase may exacerbate low back pain, deteriorate your spine and pelvis, and weaken your abdominal muscles. All of these might affect your posture.

- Put on comfortable, low-heeled shoes: For instance, walking improperly while wearing high heels might result in you losing your equilibrium. Your posture will be harmed, and your muscles will be under more stress.

- Make sure work surfaces are at a comfortable height for you, whether you're eating, cooking, or just sitting in front of a computer.

How can I sit more properly?

Many Americans spend a lot of time sitting down at home, work, or school. It's important to sit properly and stand up often to stretch:

- Frequent changes in a sitting position.

- Walk briefly around your home or place of work.

- Gently stretching your muscles on occasion can help to minimize muscular tension.

- Avoid crossing your legs and keep your ankles in front of your knees.

- Use a footrest if it isn't possible to keep your feet on the ground.

- Your shoulders shouldn't be hunched or dragged back; they should be loose.

- Keep your elbows in a close posture. The curve should be between 90 and 120 degrees.

- Support your back to the utmost degree feasible. Use a back cushion or another kind of back support if the backrest of your chair cannot accommodate your lower back's curve.

- Check to see whether your hips and thighs are supported. Your sitting position should be comfortable and your thighs and hips should be parallel to the floor.

How can I stand more erect?

- Become tall and erect.
- Your shoulders should be straight
- Make a stomach indent.
- Distribute your weight over the balls of your feet.
- Maintain a straight back.
- Naturally, your arms should hang at your sides.
- Keep your feet apart by shoulder width.

With little work, you can improve your posture; you'll look and feel better.

Regular Exercise and Stretching

Regular physical exercise is essential for keeping a flexible and healthy back. Exercise helps to improve posture, strengthen the muscles that support the spine, and maintain general spinal health. Include low-impact aerobic workouts in your program, such as cycling, swimming, or walking. Additionally, targeted back workouts like core strengthening exercises and stretching routines might be beneficial for enhancing results.

Ergonomics at Home and Work

Back health demands that ergonomic settings be created at home and the office. Your back will be properly supported and positioned throughout activities if ergonomics is done correctly. Pay attention to how your computer, chair, and desk are set up at work. Use lumbar support-equipped ergonomic seats, set your computer screen to eye level, and sit with proper posture. Make sure your sleeping surface is comfy and supportive at home by selecting furniture that offers enough support.

Weight Control

A healthy weight must be maintained if the back is to be less stressed. Weight gain may put stress on the spine, putting more strain on the discs and joints and perhaps causing back discomfort. Adopting a nutritious diet and doing regular exercise will help you reach and maintain a healthy weight, which lowers your chance of developing back discomfort and its problems.

The Value of a Healthy Diet

A healthy diet significantly contributes to overall well-being, which includes spinal health. Eat a healthy, balanced diet that is high in whole grains, lean meats, and fruits and vegetables. Concentrate on consuming foods that are rich in calcium and vitamin D, which are crucial elements for bone health. These vitamins and minerals promote healthy bones and lower the chance of diseases like osteoporosis, which may worsen back discomfort.

Avoiding Excessive Back Strain

Acute or persistent discomfort might be the consequence of too much back strain. It's essential to use good body mechanics and lifting methods to avoid strain. Avoid twisting actions, maintain the burden close to your body, and use your legs to raise heavy things rather than your back. To prevent overexertion, repeated tasks should be done for extended periods with frequent rests and position changes.

Stress Management Techniques

Back discomfort and muscular strain are both exacerbated by stress. Back pain may be relieved and stress levels can be lowered by using stress management practices. Investigate relaxing pursuits like yoga, deep breathing techniques, mindfulness meditation, and many other activities. These methods for stress management may help you have a healthy, pain-free back.

You may get several advantages by implementing these preventative steps and lifestyle modifications, including:

- Decreased chance of back discomfort and problems connected to it
- Improved back muscular flexibility and strength
- Improved alignment of the spine and posture
- Improved general health and quality of life

Chapter Five

Psychological and Emotional Well-being

Your psychological and emotional health may suffer if you have persistent back pain, in addition to your physical health. You must prioritize your psychological and emotional well-being as part of your back pain treatments and address the mind-body link. You may enhance your general well-being and quality of life by comprehending how chronic pain affects your mental health, learning pain coping mechanisms, and putting stress management and relaxation practices into practice.

The Mind-Body Connection

Because the mind and body are intertwined, chronic pain may have a profound effect on your mental and emotional health. It's critical to understand how the psychological components of pain might affect how you feel and perceive back pain. You may start addressing the emotional and psychological issues that could be causing your discomfort after you have a better grasp of the mind-body relationship.

Although managing and reducing the effects of chronic pain on your everyday life might be difficult, there are helpful coping mechanisms you can use. Among such coping mechanisms are:

Mindfulness

You may improve your outlook and lessen the mental suffering related to chronic pain by embracing your pain without passing judgment on it. Deep breathing exercises and other mindfulness techniques may help you remain present and better manage your discomfort.

(CBT) Cognitive Behavioral Therapy

The main goal of CBT is to recognize and alter unfavorable thinking patterns and behaviors related to chronic pain. Your capacity to control pain and lessen emotional suffering may be improved by confronting limiting beliefs and adopting new coping mechanisms.

Programs for Pain Management

You may get knowledge, support, and useful tools to help you deal with chronic pain by taking part in pain management programs, either alone or in a group environment. These programs often include a variety of strategies, including goal-setting, relaxation exercises, and instruction on the neurobiology of pain.

Techniques for Relaxation and Stress Management

Stress may heighten levels of chronic pain, and chronic pain itself can be made worse by stress. Exercises for relaxation and stress reduction may be used to assist break this pattern and advance emotional well-being. Think about the following methods:

Restorative Practices

To generate a state of relaxation and lessen the muscular tension brought on by pain, try deep breathing techniques, progressive muscle relaxation, or guided imagery.

Mindfulness and Meditation

Practice mindfulness meditation to develop an uncritical awareness of the present moment. By shifting your attention away from the discomfort, mindfulness may help you feel less stressed and anxious.

Investigate methods for reducing stress including taking up a hobby, spending time in nature, listening to music, keeping a diary, or doing yoga. These pursuits may serve as a vehicle for emotional release and foster a feeling of serenity and well-being.

You may improve your general well-being and your capacity to manage and live with chronic pain by addressing the psychological and emotional elements of back pain. It is crucial to seek assistance from medical personnel, psychiatrists, or pain management experts who can direct you in creating a specialized strategy to handle your particular requirements.

Keep in mind that controlling chronic pain requires a comprehensive strategy that takes into account not just the physical elements but also the psychological and emotional ones. You may develop resilience, reclaim control over your life, and enhance your general well-being by implementing these techniques into your back pain treatments.

Chapter Six

Conclusion

You have made a huge step in regaining control over your back health and reclaiming a life free from the restrictions of pain by reading our complete guide on back pain treatments. We have looked at a variety of approaches, methods, and lifestyle changes that may successfully treat back pain and encourage better, pain-free living throughout this book.

The advantages of putting your back health first and keeping it that way are transformational. Here are some of the main benefits you might anticipate:

Enhanced Physical Function: You may restore spine strength, flexibility, and mobility by using back pain remedies. You may resume activities you used to like, such as playing sports, taking long walks, or just carrying out everyday duties, with improved physical function.

Increased Quality of Life: Having chronic back pain may hurt your general health and reduce your pleasure in life. You may significantly improve your quality of life by implementing the suggestions made in this book. Greater feelings of contentment and happiness may result from the freedom from discomfort to participate in activities, pursue interests, and build meaningful connections.

Greater Freedom: Back discomfort might limit your freedom and make you dependent on other people for help. Your back pain may be actively treated and managed, allowing you to reclaim your autonomy and self-reliance. With your newfound independence, you may live your life without constraints or the need for ongoing help.

Future Problems: Investing in back pain remedies not only helps with present agony but also aids in averting future issues. You may dramatically lower your chance of experiencing new or recurring episodes of back pain by adopting healthy lifestyle choices, keeping a healthy weight, exercising often, and practicing excellent posture, protecting your long-term back health.

Psychiatric and Emotional Health:
Beyond only providing physical comfort, treating back pain has a great influence on your mental and emotional health. You will feel less emotional discomfort and have a more positive attitude toward life as you practice mindfulness, stress management, and coping skills. This

increased mental toughness supports general health and a more upbeat outlook.

Keep in mind that sustaining excellent back health requires continual dedication. It calls for perseverance, commitment, and a proactive attitude toward your well-being. Be patient on the trip and use the information and strategies in this book in your everyday activities. You may get a strong and pain-free back with perseverance, hard work, and the appropriate attitude.

Accepting back pain treatments allows you to live a life of liberty, pleasure, and well-being. You may regain control of your body and enable yourself to enjoy life to the fullest by taking responsibility for your back health. So, go off on your road to a better, happier, and pain-free future with confidence and the solutions described in this book.

Shelby A. Nicholson, MD   61

Wishing you a life full of energy and fortitude
as you continue to put your back health first.
You deserve it.

Shelby A. Nicholson, MD   62